Anti-Inflammatory Diet Cookbook for Beginners

Nourish Your Body, Fight Inflammation, and Embrace Wellness with Flavorful Recipes

By

Evelyn C. Hill

Table of Contents

CHAPTER 4: LUNCH RECIPES

CHAPTER 5: DINNER RECIPES

CHAPTER 6: SNACKS AND APPETIZERS RECIPES

Dairy-Free Banana Ice Cream

Vegan Lentil Stew

Low-Sugar Coconut Macaroons

Gluten-Free Sweet Potato Pancakes

Dairy-Free Green Smoothie Bowl

CONCLUSION

Introduction

Inflammation is a normal process that allows your body to heal and fight itself against injury. However, persistent inflammation can cause a variety of health problems, including heart disease, diabetes, arthritis, and even certain malignancies. The good news is that by making smart dietary changes, you may help control and minimize inflammation, so improving your overall health and wellbeing.

Inflammation is your body's way of protecting itself against infection, disease, and injury. When your cells are under trouble, they emit molecules that signal your immune system. This causes an inflammatory reaction, which brings more blood to the injured area, as well as immune cells and hormones that aid in the healing of damaged tissue. While this process is necessary for healing, prolonged inflammation can cause problems. Unlike acute inflammation, which is a temporary response, chronic inflammation persists, emitting inflammatory chemicals even when there is no visible threat.

An anti-inflammatory diet emphasizes nutrient-dense foods that reduce inflammation and promote general health. Incorporating a mix of fruits, vegetables, whole grains, lean proteins, and healthy fats into your meals helps supply your body with the nutrition it requires to combat inflammation. This diet has been demonstrated to increase energy levels, improve digestion, aid in weight management, and lower the risk of chronic diseases.

The anti-inflammatory diet is not limited to people who currently have chronic inflammation. It's an effective strategy for everyone trying to improve their health and avoid disease. Whether you have an autoimmune problem, chronic pain, or simply want to enhance your general health, this diet can provide various benefits. It's also a wonderful approach to boost your immune system and live a healthier, more active lifestyle.

Chapter 1

What is Inflammation?

Inflammation is a complex biological response that acts as the body's defense against harmful stimuli such viruses, injuries, and irritants. It is an essential component of the immune system's reaction to keep tissues stable and promote healing.

Acute versus Chronic Inflammation

Acute inflammation: This is the body's initial reaction to an injury or infection. It is distinguished by redness, heat, swelling, discomfort, and loss of function at the point of damage. For example, when you cut your finger, the body sends white blood cells to the injury site to combat infection and start the healing process. This form of inflammation is usually only present for a few days.

Chronic inflammation. In contrast to acute inflammation, chronic inflammation is a sluggish, long-term response that might last months or even years. It happens when the body's inflammatory reaction fails to resolve the issue or accidentally targets healthy tissues. Chronic inflammation is linked to a variety of conditions, including heart disease, diabetes, arthritis, and certain malignancies. Chronic inflammation can be caused by a poor diet, a lack of exercise, stress, or exposure to environmental contaminants.

The Inflammatory Response

1. Inflammation starts when the body perceives a threat, such as infection by bacteria, viruses, or pathogens, or tissue damage from injury or trauma. Immune cells, such as macrophages and dendritic cells, sense these dangers and produce signaling chemicals known as cytokines.

2. Cytokines widen blood vessels in the affected area, boosting blood flow and facilitating immune cell, antibody, and nutrition delivery to the site of inflammation. Blood artery permeability also increases, allowing fluid, proteins, and immune cells to flow from the bloodstream to the surrounding tissue.

3. Migration of Immune Cells: White blood cells, such as neutrophils and monocytes, migrate to the site of inflammation. These immune cells help to combat pathogens, remove damaged cells and debris, and initiate tissue repair.

4. Activation of Immune Response: Immune cells produce more cytokines and inflammatory mediators, like prostaglandins and leukotrienes, amplifying the inflammatory response. This mechanism serves to confine and eradicate the threat while also encouraging tissue repair and regeneration.

5. Resolution and Healing: Once a threat is neutralized, regulatory T cells and anti-inflammatory cytokines assist reduce inflammation. The resolution phase entails removing inflammatory cells and supporting tissue healing in order to restore normal function.

Types of Inflammation

1. Acute inflammation is a short-term response to tissue injury, infection, or trauma. Acute inflammation is distinguished by localized redness, swelling, heat, discomfort, and loss of functionality. It is a defense mechanism that aids in the elimination of infections, the removal of damaged cells, and the initiation of tissue repair.

2. Chronic Inflammation: This low-grade inflammatory state can linger for weeks, months, or even years. It can be caused by unresolved acute inflammation, autoimmune illnesses, chronic infections, or persistent exposure to irritants (such smoking or obesity). Chronic inflammation can lead to the development of a variety of diseases, including cardiovascular disease, diabetes, arthritis, and several malignancies.

Common Causes of Inflammation

Several things can cause inflammation, such as:

1. Infections: Bacterial, viral, or fungal infections can result in acute or chronic inflammation.

2. Physical injuries such as cuts, scratches, or burns may cause acute inflammation.

3. Toxins: Environmental toxins, pollutants, or chemicals may cause inflammation.

4. Unhealthy Diet: Consuming sweets, processed carbs, and unhealthy fats can increase inflammation.

5. Chronic stress can increase cortisol and other stress chemicals, causing inflammation.

6. Autoimmune Disorders: Rheumatoid arthritis and lupus occur when the immune system erroneously attacks the body's own tissues, resulting in chronic inflammation.

Advantages of an Anti-inflammatory Diet

Adopting an anti-inflammatory diet can have a significant impact on overall health and wellness. This diet focuses on complete, nutrient-dense meals that reduce inflammation and promote the body's natural healing processes.

• Improved energy levels.

A diet high in anti-inflammatory foods can help regulate blood sugar and minimize energy crashes. Whole grains, lean proteins, and healthy fats provide all-day energy, minimizing weariness and improving mental clarity.

• Enhanced digestive health.

Anti-inflammatory meals are often strong in fiber, which improves proper digestion and bowel motions. A well-balanced diet rich in fruits, vegetables, and whole grains will help to maintain a healthy gut microbiome and reduce symptoms of bloating, gas, and constipation.

• Improved Weight Management.

Chronic inflammation is commonly associated with weight gain and obesity. Reducing inflammation allows the body to better regulate metabolism and maintain a healthy weight. Anti-inflammatory foods have less calories and more nutrients, making it easier to maintain a healthy weight without feeling deprived.

• Reduced risk of chronic diseases.

An anti-inflammatory diet can help reduce your chance of acquiring chronic diseases including heart disease, diabetes, and some malignancies. Foods high in antioxidants, vitamins, and minerals counteract oxidative stress and protect the body's cells from harm.

• Relief of chronic pain.

An anti-inflammatory diet can assist people with arthritis and other inflammatory disorders reduce pain and improve mobility. Anti-inflammatory foods can reduce the severity of symptoms and improve quality of life.

• Improved mental health.

Chronic inflammation has been linked to a variety of mental health issues, including sadness and anxiety. An anti-inflammatory diet high in omega-3 fatty acids, antioxidants, and other brain-boosting foods can help improve mental health and cognitive function.

• Stronger immune system.

By lowering inflammation, the immune system can work more effectively. This means improved infection resistance and faster recovery from illness. Anti-inflammatory foods including leafy greens, berries, and nuts are high in vitamins and minerals that improve immune function.

Choosing an anti-inflammatory diet is a significant step toward achieving and maintaining good health. You can live a healthy, disease-free life by eating complete, natural foods and avoiding those that cause inflammation.

Who Could Benefit From This Diet?

The anti-inflammatory diet is a varied and healthy eating plan that can benefit a wide spectrum of people. Whether you are suffering with specific health difficulties or simply want to improve your overall well-being, this diet has many benefits. An anti-inflammatory diet can be particularly beneficial to the following groups of people:

People with chronic inflammatory conditions

Arthritis and joint pain. Rheumatoid arthritis and osteoarthritis are both characterized by chronic joint inflammation. An anti-inflammatory diet can help to relieve pain and stiffness, improve joint function, and potentially decrease the progression of certain illnesses. Foods high in omega-3 fatty acids, such as fatty fish, flaxseeds, and walnuts, are especially beneficial to joint health.

Autoimmune Disorders: An anti-inflammatory diet can help those suffering from autoimmune disorders like lupus, multiple sclerosis, and inflammatory bowel disease (IBD). This diet, which reduces systemic inflammation, can help control symptoms and enhance quality of life. Anti-inflammatory foods such as leafy greens, berries, and turmeric can boost immune health and minimize flare-ups.

Cardiovascular Health: Chronic inflammation increases the risk of heart disease and stroke. An anti-inflammatory diet that includes fruits, vegetables, whole grains, and healthy fats can help lower blood pressure, cholesterol, and the risk of heart disease. Olive oil, almonds, and fatty seafood are especially heart-healthy.

Metabolic Health

Diabetes and Insulin Resistance: Inflammation is a key factor in the development of insulin resistance and type 2 diabetes. An anti-inflammatory diet can help regulate blood sugar, enhance insulin sensitivity, and lower the risk of diabetes complications. Fiber-rich meals such as whole grains, lentils, and non-starchy vegetables can help efficiently control blood sugar levels.

Mental Health and Cognitive Function

Depression and Anxiety: New research indicates a relationship between chronic inflammation and mental health issues like depression and anxiety. An anti-inflammatory diet high in antioxidants and omega-3 fatty acids can boost brain health and mood. Foods with brain-boosting characteristics include salmon, blueberries, and dark leafy greens.

Inflammation is linked to cognitive impairment and neurodegenerative illnesses such as Alzheimer's. An anti-inflammatory diet can help to maintain brain health and lower the risk of cognitive impairment. Antioxidant-rich foods including berries, almonds, and seeds are especially good for sustaining cognitive function.

Digestive Health: IBS and other digestive disorders. Chronic inflammation in the gut can cause a variety of digestive problems, including IBS, Crohn's disease, and ulcerative colitis. An anti-inflammatory diet can help to calm the digestive system, alleviate symptoms, and support a healthy gut microbiota. Fermented foods such as yogurt, kefir, and sauerkraut, as well as fiber-rich fruits and vegetables, are great for gut health.

Skin Health

Eczema, psoriasis, and acne: Eczema, psoriasis, and acne are among skin diseases that are commonly associated with inflammation. An anti-inflammatory diet can help to reduce skin inflammation, enhance skin health, and minimize the number and severity of flare-ups. Avocados, almonds, and green tea are examples of foods high in antioxidants and good fats that can benefit skin health.

General well-being and healthy aging: Inflammation can speed up the aging process and contribute to age-related disorders. An anti-inflammatory diet can promote healthy aging by lowering oxidative stress and improving cellular health. A longevity-focused diet includes nutrient-dense foods such as colorful fruits and vegetables, healthy grains, and lean proteins.

Weight Management: Chronic inflammation is frequently associated with obesity and problems decreasing weight. An anti-inflammatory diet, which emphasizes whole, unprocessed foods, can aid in weight reduction and maintenance by lowering inflammation, boosting metabolism, and increasing satiety. Incorporating a range of nutrient-dense foods ensures that you obtain enough vitamins and minerals for good health.

An anti-inflammatory diet is an effective technique that can help a wide spectrum of people. Whether you want to manage a chronic disease, improve your mental and cognitive health, improve your digestive and skin health, or simply promote general well-being, this diet provides a sustainable and beneficial way of eating. Focusing on anti-inflammatory foods allows you to take proactive measures toward a healthier, more vibrant existence.

Getting Started: Understanding the Anti-Inflammatory Diet.

The anti-inflammatory diet is intended to minimize chronic inflammation, which can lead to a variety of health conditions. This diet emphasizes entire, nutrient-dense meals while limiting or eliminating those that can cause inflammation.

Key Principles

1. Focus on Whole Foods: Prioritize fresh, unprocessed foods. Whole foods are high in critical nutrients and include no added sweets, harmful fats, or artificial substances.

2. Create a beautiful platter with a variety of fruits and vegetables. These foods are high in antioxidants, vitamins, and minerals, all of which assist to reduce inflammation.

3. Choose Healthy Fats: Consume healthy fats like olive oil, avocados, almonds, and seeds. Omega-3 fatty acids, found in fatty fish such as salmon and flaxseed, are very advantageous.

4. Replace processed grains with whole grains, such as brown rice, quinoa, and wheat. Whole grains contain fiber, which aids digestion and lowers inflammation.

5. Consume lean proteins, like poultry, fish, beans, and lentils. Plant-based proteins are effective at reducing inflammation.

6. Limit processed foods. Avoid processed and packaged foods that have extra sugars, bad fats, and artificial ingredients.

7. Stay Hydrated: Drink plenty of water and consume anti-inflammatory beverages such as green tea and herbal teas.

Essential Kitchen Tools

The correct kitchen gadgets can make making anti-inflammatory meals simpler and more fun. Here are some important things to consider:

1. Invest in a good knife set. To chop, slice, and dice items, you'll need a sharp chef's knife, a paring knife, and a serrated knife.

2. Use separate chopping boards for meat and vegetables to avoid cross-contamination.

3. Invest in non-toxic, non-stick cookware, including stainless steel, cast iron, or ceramic pots and pans.

4. Blender/Food Processor: Ideal for preparing smoothies, soups, sauces, and chopping items.

5. Measuring Cups and Spoons: Accurate measures aid in recipe preparation and portion control.

6. Mixing Bowls: Available in various sizes to combine ingredients and prepare dishes.

7. Use baking sheets and pans to roast veggies, bake fish, and prepare healthful snacks.

8. Storage Containers: Use glass or BPA-free plastic containers to store leftovers and prepared items.

Stocking Your Pantry

A well-stocked pantry is essential for following an anti-inflammatory diet. Here is a list of basics to have on hand:

Grains and Legumes

- Quinoa

- Brown Rice

- Oats

- Barley

- Lentils

- Chickpeas

- Black Beans

Nuts and Seeds

- Almonds

- Walnuts

- Chia Seeds

- Flaxseeds

- Pumpkin Seeds

- Sunflower Seeds

Healthy Fats and Oils

- Extra Virgin Olive Oil

- Coconut Oil

- Avocado Oil

- Nut Butters (e.g., almond butter, peanut butter)

Herbs and Spices

- Turmeric

- Ginger

- Garlic Powder

- Cinnamon

- Cumin

- Paprika

- Basil

- Oregano

Condiments and Sauces

- Low-Sodium Soy Sauce or Tamari

- Apple Cider Vinegar

- Balsamic Vinegar

- Honey or Maple Syrup (in moderation)

- Mustard

Canned and Packaged Goods

- Tomatoes (diced, crushed, or pureed)

- Broths and Stocks (preferably low-sodium)

- Tuna or Salmon (packed in water)

Fresh and Frozen Produce

- Leafy Greens (e.g., spinach, kale)

- Berries (fresh or frozen)

- Cruciferous Vegetables (e.g., broccoli, cauliflower)

- Citrus Fruits (e.g., lemons, oranges)

- Root Vegetables (e.g., carrots, sweet potatoes)

Beverages

- Green Tea

- Herbal Teas

- Filtered Water

Understanding the fundamentals of the anti-inflammatory diet, equipping your kitchen with the necessary tools, and stocking your pantry with important foods all lay the groundwork for a successful road to improved health. This preparation will make it easier to prepare tasty, healthy meals that reduce inflammation and promote general health.

Chapter 2

The Role of Diet in Inflammation

Diet plays an important function in controlling inflammation in the body. Certain foods can either increase or decrease inflammation, making dietary choices an important component in controlling chronic inflammatory disorders and maintaining general health.

How Food Can Cause Inflammation

1. Processed foods are heavy in added sugars, harmful fats (e.g. trans and saturated fats), processed carbs, and artificial additives. These components may cause inflammation and contribute to chronic health issues such as obesity, diabetes, and cardiovascular disease.

2. Refined Carbohydrates: Consuming white bread, pastries, sugary snacks, and drinks can promote fast blood sugar increases, resulting in increased production of inflammatory molecules like cytokines. A high-refined-carbohydrate diet can lead to insulin resistance and systemic inflammation.

3. Trans fats, commonly found in partly hydrogenated oils used in fried foods, baked products, and processed snacks, can cause inflammation and raise the risk of heart disease. Avoiding trans fats is critical for keeping a good inflammatory balance.

4. Excess Sugar: Consuming too much sugar, particularly high-fructose corn syrup and added sugars in processed foods and beverages, can cause chronic low-grade inflammation. Sugar can also cause insulin resistance, weight gain, and metabolic diseases.

5. Unhealthy fats. Saturated fats, which are found in red meat, full-fat dairy products, and some oils such as palm oil and coconut oil, can cause inflammation if ingested in excess. Instead, eat healthier fats like monounsaturated fats (found in olive oil, avocados, and almonds) and omega-3 fatty acids (found in fish, flaxseeds, and walnuts).

6. Food Allergies and Sensitivities: Some people may be sensitive or allergic to particular foods, such as gluten, dairy, soy, or nightshade vegetables. Consuming

certain trigger foods might cause immunological responses and inflammation in vulnerable people.

Anti-inflammatory Nutrients

On the other hand, many nutrients found in whole, unprocessed foods have anti-inflammatory effects. Adding these nutrients to your diet can help reduce inflammation and improve overall health:

1. Omega-3 Fatty Acids: Found in fatty fish (e.g. salmon, sardines, mackerel), flaxseeds, chia seeds, and walnuts, omega-3 fatty acids have powerful anti-inflammatory properties. They can help reduce the amounts of inflammatory chemicals such as cytokines and prostaglandin.

2. Fruits, vegetables, nuts, and seeds contain antioxidants that neutralize free radicals and minimize oxidative stress, a common cause of inflammation. Berries, dark leafy greens, bell peppers, and tomatoes are all good sources of antioxidants.

3. Polyphenols: Plant chemicals possess anti-inflammatory and antioxidant capabilities. They are commonly found in foods such as green tea, olive oil, dark chocolate, and colorful fruits and vegetables.

4. Dietary fiber from whole grains, legumes, fruits, and vegetables promotes intestinal health and decreases inflammation. Fiber-rich diets also help to control blood sugar levels and increase satiety.

5. Vitamins and minerals can reduce inflammation and improve immunological function. Citrus fruits, bell peppers, and strawberries are good sources of vitamin C; nuts, seeds, and spinach are good sources of vitamin E; and leafy greens, almonds, and whole grains contain magnesium.

Turmeric, a spice widely used in curry foods, includes curcumin, a molecule with powerful anti-inflammatory properties. Adding turmeric to your meals or taking curcumin pills can help reduce inflammation.

Understanding how different foods can promote or reduce inflammation allows you to make more informed dietary choices that benefit your overall health and well-being. Incorporating anti-inflammatory foods into your diet and avoiding inflammatory triggers can help control chronic inflammation and lower your risk of linked health problems.

Foods to Eat and Avoid on an Anti-Inflamatory Diet

Making conscious food selections is essential while following an anti-inflammatory diet. By eating anti-inflammatory foods and avoiding pro-inflammatory ones, you can help reduce chronic inflammation, strengthen your immune system, and improve general health and well-being.

Foods To Eat

1. Fruits and vegetables:

• Berries: Blueberries, strawberries, raspberries, and blackberries contain antioxidants and phytochemicals that reduce inflammation.

• Leafy greens such as spinach, kale, Swiss chard, and collard greens have high levels of vitamins, minerals, and antioxidants.

• Colorful vegetables, such as bell peppers, tomatoes, carrots, beets, and sweet potatoes, provide various nutrients and anti-inflammatory chemicals.

2. Whole Grains: • Quinoa is a gluten-free grain rich in protein, fiber, and important minerals.

• Brown rice is high in fiber and antioxidants, which improve digestive health and reduce inflammation.

• Oats include beta-glucans, which offer anti-inflammatory and immune-boosting benefits.

3. Healthy Fats: • Fatty Fish: Salmon, sardines, trout, and mackerel contain omega-3 fatty acids, which have powerful anti-inflammatory properties.

• Avocados include monounsaturated fats, vitamins, and minerals, which promote heart health and reduce inflammation.

• Nuts and seeds: Almonds, walnuts, flaxseeds, chia seeds, and hemp seeds include healthful fats, fiber, and antioxidants.

4. Lean protein:

• Skinless chicken and turkey are lean protein sources with essential amino acids and low saturated fat.

• Legumes, including beans, lentils, chickpeas, and peas, are high in fiber, vitamins, and minerals.

5. Herbs & spices.

• Turmeric contains curcumin, a powerful anti-inflammatory substance with antioxidant effects.

• Ginger has anti-inflammatory and digestive properties and is widely used in teas, stir-fries, and soups.

• Garlic contains allicin, which has immune-boosting and anti-inflammatory properties.

6. Healthy Beverages: • Green tea contains antioxidants called catechins, which have anti-inflammatory and health-promoting qualities.

• Herbal teas such as chamomile, peppermint, and ginger offer relaxing and anti-inflammatory properties.

Foods to avoid.

1. Processed and Sugary Foods: • Sodas and Sugary Drinks: Contain added sugars, which can cause inflammation and metabolic issues.

Excessive sugar consumption can cause inflammation, insulin resistance, and weight gain.

• Processed foods like chips, cookies, and pastries can include unhealthy fats, sugars, and additives.

2. Trans Fats: • Deep-fried meals (e.g., french fries, fried chicken, and doughnuts) contain trans fats, which can cause inflammation and heart disease.

• Commercially baked items with partially hydrogenated oils often include trans fats.

3. Refined Carbohydrates: • White Bread and Pastries: Refined grains lack fiber and can increase blood sugar levels, causing inflammation and insulin resistance.

• Choose whole grains, such as brown rice, rather processed white rice.

4. Processed Meats: • Hot dogs, sausages, bacon, and deli meats may contain preservatives, sodium, and unhealthy fats that can cause inflammation and increase disease risk.

5. Excessive Alcohol: • Heavy drinking can cause liver inflammation and contribute to chronic health issues.

6. Artificial Additives: • Artificial Sweeteners: Certain artificial sweeteners might cause inflammation and alter gut health in sensitive individuals.

• Processed foods with artificial flavors and colors may trigger inflammation and allergies in certain individuals.

An anti-inflammatory diet emphasizes complete, nutrient-dense foods that reduce inflammation and promote general health. A balanced and inflammation-fighting eating plan can be created by focusing on fruits and vegetables, whole grains, healthy fats, lean proteins, and anti-inflammatory herbs and spices while avoiding processed meals, sweets, bad fats, and artificial chemicals. It is critical to listen to your body and make nutritional decisions that promote health and energy.

Chapter 3: Breakfast Recipes

Turmeric Oatmeal

- **Prep Time:** 5 minutes

- **Cook Time:** 10 minutes

- **Serving Size:** 2 servings

Ingredients:

- 1 cup rolled oats

- 2 cups water or almond milk

- 1 teaspoon turmeric powder

- 1/2 teaspoon cinnamon

- 1 tablespoon honey or maple syrup (optional)

- Fresh berries for topping

- Chopped nuts for topping

Instructions:

1. In a saucepan, bring water or almond milk to a boil.

2. Stir in the rolled oats, turmeric powder, and cinnamon.

3. Reduce heat and simmer for 5-7 minutes until the oats are cooked and creamy.

4. Sweeten with honey or maple syrup if desired.

5. Serve the oatmeal in bowls, topped with fresh berries and chopped nuts.

Nutritional Facts (per serving):

- Calories: 250 kcal

- Protein: 6g

- Carbohydrates: 44g

- Fat: 6g

- Fiber: 6g

Avocado Toast with Poached Egg

- **Prep Time:** 5 minutes

- **Cook Time:** 5 minutes

- **Serving Size:** 1 serving

Ingredients:

- 1 slice whole-grain bread

- 1/2 ripe avocado, mashed

- 1 poached egg

- Salt and pepper to taste

- Fresh herbs for garnish (optional)

Instructions:

1. Toast the whole-grain bread until golden brown.

2. Spread the mashed avocado evenly on the toast.

3. Top with a poached egg.

4. Season with salt, pepper, and fresh herbs if desired.

Nutritional Facts (per serving):

- Calories: 280 kcal

- Protein: 13g

- Carbohydrates: 20g

- Fat: 18g

- Fiber: 9g

Berry Smoothie Bowl

- **Prep Time:** 5 minutes

- **Cook Time:** 0 minutes

- **Serving Size:** 1 serving

Ingredients:

- 1 cup mixed berries (strawberries, blueberries, raspberries)

- 1/2 ripe banana

- 1/2 cup almond milk

- 1 tablespoon chia seeds

- 1 tablespoon almond butter

- Toppings: sliced almonds, shredded coconut, fresh berries

Instructions:

1. In a blender, combine the mixed berries, banana, almond milk, chia seeds, and almond butter.

2. Blend until smooth and creamy.

3. Pour the smoothie into a bowl.

4. Top with sliced almonds, shredded coconut, and fresh berries.

Nutritional Facts (per serving):

- Calories: 320 kcal

- Protein: 8g

- Carbohydrates: 35g

- Fat: 18g

- Fiber: 12g

Chia Seed Pudding

- **Prep Time:** 5 minutes (+chilling time)

- **Cook Time:** 0 minutes

- **Serving Size:** 2 servings

Ingredients:

- 1/4 cup chia seeds

- 1 cup almond milk

- 1 tablespoon honey or maple syrup

- 1/2 teaspoon vanilla extract

- Fresh fruit for topping

Instructions:

1. In a bowl, whisk together chia seeds, almond milk, honey or maple syrup, and vanilla extract.

2. Cover and refrigerate for at least 2 hours or overnight until the mixture thickens.

3. Stir the chia seed pudding before serving.

4. Top with fresh fruit of your choice.

Nutritional Facts (per serving):

- Calories: 180 kcal

- Protein: 4g

- Carbohydrates: 20g

- Fat: 9g

- Fiber: 10g

Spinach and Mushroom Omelette

- **Prep Time:** 5 minutes

- **Cook Time:** 10 minutes

- **Serving Size:** 1 serving

Ingredients:

- 2 large eggs

- 1 cup fresh spinach, chopped

- 1/2 cup mushrooms, sliced

- 1/4 cup diced onions

- 1 tablespoon olive oil

- Salt and pepper to taste

- Fresh herbs for garnish (optional)

Instructions:

1. In a skillet, heat olive oil over medium heat.

2. Add onions and mushrooms, sauté until softened.

3. Add chopped spinach and cook until wilted.

4. In a bowl, beat the eggs and season with salt and pepper.

5. Pour the beaten eggs into the skillet, covering the vegetables evenly.

6. Cook until the omelette is set, then fold it in half.

7. Garnish with fresh herbs if desired.

Nutritional Facts (per serving):

- Calories: 290 kcal

- Protein: 17g

- Carbohydrates: 6g

- Fat: 22g

- Fiber: 2g

Greek Yogurt Parfait

- **Prep Time:** 5 minutes

- **Cook Time:** 0 minutes

- **Serving Size:** 1 serving

Ingredients:

- 1 cup Greek yogurt (unsweetened)

- 1/2 cup mixed berries (strawberries, blueberries)

- 1 tablespoon honey or maple syrup

- 2 tablespoons granola

- Chopped nuts for topping (optional)

Instructions:

1. In a glass or bowl, layer Greek yogurt, mixed berries, and granola.

2. Drizzle honey or maple syrup over the layers.

3. Repeat the layers if desired.

4. Top with chopped nuts for added crunch.

Nutritional Facts (per serving):

- Calories: 320 kcal

- Protein: 20g

- Carbohydrates: 40g

- Fat: 10g

- Fiber: 6g

Sweet Potato Hash

- **Prep Time:** 10 minutes

- **Cook Time:** 20 minutes

- **Serving Size:** 2 servings

Ingredients:

- 2 medium sweet potatoes, peeled and diced

- 1 bell pepper, diced

- 1 small onion, diced

- 2 tablespoons olive oil

- 1 teaspoon paprika

- Salt and pepper to taste

- Fresh parsley for garnish (optional)

Instructions:

1. In a skillet, heat olive oil over medium heat.

2. Add diced sweet potatoes and cook until slightly browned and softened.

3. Add diced bell pepper and onion to the skillet.

4. Season with paprika, salt, and pepper.

5. Cook until vegetables are tender and flavorful.

6. Garnish with fresh parsley before serving.

Nutritional Facts (per serving):

- Calories: 250 kcal

- Protein: 3g

- Carbohydrates: 30g

- Fat: 14g

- Fiber: 5g

Almond Flour Pancakes

- **Prep Time:** 10 minutes

- **Cook Time:** 10 minutes

- **Serving Size:** 2 servings

Ingredients:

- 1 cup almond flour

- 2 large eggs

- 1/2 cup almond milk

- 1 tablespoon honey or maple syrup

- 1 teaspoon baking powder

- 1/2 teaspoon vanilla extract

- Pinch of salt

- Fresh berries for topping

Instructions:

1. In a bowl, whisk together almond flour, eggs, almond milk, honey or maple syrup, baking powder, vanilla extract, and salt until smooth.

2. Heat a non-stick skillet or griddle over medium heat.

3. Pour batter onto the skillet to form pancakes.

4. Cook until bubbles form on the surface, then flip and cook until golden brown.

5. Serve the pancakes topped with fresh berries.

Nutritional Facts (per serving):

- Calories: 350 kcal

- Protein: 12g

- Carbohydrates: 20g

- Fat: 25g

- Fiber: 5g

Green Shakshuka

- **Prep Time:** 10 minutes

- **Cook Time:** 20 minutes

- **Serving Size:** 2 servings

Ingredients:

- 4 large eggs

- 2 cups fresh spinach

- 1 cup kale, chopped

- 1 bell pepper, diced

- 1/2 onion, diced
- 2 cloves garlic, minced
- 1 tablespoon olive oil
- 1 teaspoon cumin
- Salt and pepper to taste
- Feta cheese for topping (optional)

Instructions:

1. In a skillet, heat olive oil over medium heat.
2. Sauté diced onion and bell pepper until softened.
3. Add minced garlic and chopped kale to the skillet.
4. Stir in cumin, salt, and pepper.
5. Add fresh spinach and cook until wilted.
6. Create wells in the vegetable mixture and crack eggs into each well.
7. Cover the skillet and cook until eggs are set to your desired doneness.
8. Sprinkle with crumbled feta cheese before serving.

Nutritional Facts (per serving):

- Calories: 280 kcal
- Protein: 16g
- Carbohydrates: 12g
- Fat: 18g
- Fiber: 5g

Coconut Chia Seed Pudding

- **Prep Time:** 5 minutes (+chilling time)

- **Cook Time:** 0 minutes

- **Serving Size:** 2 servings

Ingredients:

- 1/4 cup chia seeds

- 1 cup coconut milk (unsweetened)

- 1 tablespoon honey or maple syrup

- 1/2 teaspoon vanilla extract

- Fresh fruit for topping

- Toasted coconut flakes for garnish

Instructions:

1. In a bowl, whisk together chia seeds, coconut milk, honey or maple syrup, and vanilla extract.

2. Cover and refrigerate for at least 2 hours or overnight until the mixture thickens.

3. Stir the chia seed pudding before serving.

4. Top with fresh fruit of your choice and toasted coconut flakes.

Nutritional Facts (per serving):

- Calories: 220 kcal

- Protein: 4g

- Carbohydrates: 20g

- Fat: 15g

- Fiber: 10g

Almond Butter Banana Overnight Oats

- **Prep Time:** 5 minutes (+chilling time)
- **Cook Time:** 0 minutes
- **Serving Size:** 1 serving

Ingredients:

- 1/2 cup rolled oats
- 1/2 cup almond milk
- 1 tablespoon almond butter
- 1/2 ripe banana, mashed
- 1 tablespoon chia seeds
- 1/2 teaspoon cinnamon
- 1 teaspoon honey or maple syrup (optional)
- Sliced banana and chopped almonds for topping

Instructions:

1. In a jar or bowl, combine rolled oats, almond milk, almond butter, mashed banana, chia seeds, cinnamon, and honey or maple syrup.
2. Stir well to mix all ingredients thoroughly.
3. Cover the jar or bowl and refrigerate overnight or for at least 4 hours.
4. Before serving, stir the overnight oats and add a splash of almond milk if desired.
5. Top with sliced banana and chopped almonds.

Nutritional Facts (per serving):

- Calories: 380 kcal
- Protein: 10g

- Carbohydrates: 50g

- Fat: 17g

- Fiber: 9g

Veggie Egg Muffins

- **Prep Time:** 10 minutes

- **Cook Time:** 20 minutes

- **Serving Size:** 4 servings

Ingredients:

- 6 large eggs

- 1/2 cup diced bell peppers

- 1/2 cup diced tomatoes

- 1/4 cup diced onions

- 1/4 cup chopped spinach

- Salt and pepper to taste

- Olive oil for greasing muffin tin

- Fresh herbs for garnish (optional)

Instructions:

1. Preheat oven to 350°F (175°C) and grease a muffin tin with olive oil.

2. In a bowl, whisk together eggs, diced bell peppers, tomatoes, onions, chopped spinach, salt, and pepper.

3. Pour the egg mixture into the greased muffin tin, filling each cup about 3/4 full.

4. Bake in the preheated oven for 15-20 minutes or until the egg muffins are set and lightly golden.

5. Allow the egg muffins to cool slightly before removing them from the muffin tin.

6. Garnish with fresh herbs before serving.

Nutritional Facts (per serving, 2 egg muffins):

- Calories: 150 kcal

- Protein: 12g

- Carbohydrates: 5g

- Fat: 9g

- Fiber: 1g

Coconut Flour Pancakes

- **Prep Time:** 10 minutes

- **Cook Time:** 10 minutes

- **Serving Size:** 2 servings

Ingredients:

- 1/2 cup coconut flour

- 4 large eggs

- 1/2 cup coconut milk (unsweetened)

- 1 tablespoon honey or maple syrup

- 1 teaspoon baking powder

- 1/2 teaspoon vanilla extract

- Pinch of salt

- Fresh berries for topping

Instructions:

1. In a bowl, whisk together coconut flour, eggs, coconut milk, honey or maple syrup, baking powder, vanilla extract, and salt until smooth.

2. Heat a non-stick skillet or griddle over medium heat.

3. Pour batter onto the skillet to form pancakes.

4. Cook until bubbles form on the surface, then flip and cook until golden brown.

5. Serve the pancakes topped with fresh berries.

Nutritional Facts (per serving):

- Calories: 320 kcal

- Protein: 14g

- Carbohydrates: 20g

- Fat: 20g

- Fiber: 8g

Mediterranean Breakfast Bowl

- **Prep Time:** 10 minutes

- **Cook Time:** 10 minutes

- **Serving Size:** 2 servings

Ingredients:

- 1 cup cooked quinoa

- 4 large eggs

- 1/2 cup cherry tomatoes, halved

- 1/4 cup sliced cucumbers

- 1/4 cup crumbled feta cheese

- 2 tablespoons Kalamata olives, sliced

- 1 tablespoon olive oil

- Salt and pepper to taste

- Fresh parsley for garnish

Instructions:

1. In a skillet, heat olive oil over medium heat.

2. Crack eggs into the skillet and cook to your desired doneness (scrambled, fried, or poached).

3. In bowls, divide cooked quinoa evenly.

4. Top the quinoa with cooked eggs, cherry tomatoes, sliced cucumbers, crumbled feta cheese, and sliced Kalamata olives.

5. Season with salt, pepper, and garnish with fresh parsley.

Nutritional Facts (per serving):

- Calories: 380 kcal

- Protein: 20g

- Carbohydrates: 30g

- Fat: 20g

- Fiber: 5g

Blueberry Chia Seed Smoothie

- **Prep Time:** 5 minutes

- **Cook Time:** 0 minutes

- **Serving Size:** 1 serving

Ingredients:

- 1 cup almond milk (unsweetened)

- 1/2 cup frozen blueberries

- 1 tablespoon chia seeds

- 1 tablespoon almond butter

- 1 teaspoon honey or maple syrup (optional)

- Ice cubes (optional)

Instructions:

1. In a blender, combine almond milk, frozen blueberries, chia seeds, almond butter, and honey or maple syrup.

2. Add ice cubes if desired for a colder smoothie.

3. Blend until smooth and creamy.

4. Pour the smoothie into a glass and enjoy immediately.

Nutritional Facts (per serving):

- Calories: 250 kcal

- Protein: 6g

- Carbohydrates: 20g

- Fat: 15g

- Fiber: 8g

Chapter 4: Lunch Recipes

Quinoa and Chickpea Salad

- **Prep Time:** 15 minutes
- **Cook Time:** 15 minutes
- **Serving Size:** 4 servings

Ingredients:

- 1 cup quinoa, rinsed
- 2 cups water
- 1 can (15 oz) chickpeas, drained and rinsed
- 1 cup cherry tomatoes, halved
- 1 cucumber, diced
- 1/4 cup red onion, finely chopped
- 1/4 cup fresh parsley, chopped
- 1/4 cup fresh lemon juice
- 3 tablespoons olive oil
- Salt and pepper to taste

Instructions:

1. In a medium pot, bring quinoa and water to a boil. Reduce heat, cover, and simmer for 15 minutes or until quinoa is cooked.
2. In a large bowl, combine cooked quinoa, chickpeas, cherry tomatoes, cucumber, red onion, and parsley.
3. In a small bowl, whisk together lemon juice, olive oil, salt, and pepper.
4. Pour the dressing over the salad and toss to combine.
5. Serve immediately or refrigerate for later.

Nutritional Facts (per serving):

- Calories: 280 kcal

- Protein: 9g

- Carbohydrates: 37g

- Fat: 11g

- Fiber: 7g

Lentil and Vegetable Soup

- **Prep Time:** 10 minutes

- **Cook Time:** 30 minutes

- **Serving Size:** 4 servings

Ingredients:

- 1 cup dried lentils, rinsed

- 1 carrot, diced

- 1 celery stalk, diced

- 1 onion, diced

- 3 garlic cloves, minced

- 1 can (14.5 oz) diced tomatoes

- 6 cups vegetable broth

- 1 teaspoon cumin

- 1 teaspoon turmeric

- 1 teaspoon paprika

- Salt and pepper to taste

- 2 tablespoons olive oil

- Fresh spinach for garnish

Instructions:

1. In a large pot, heat olive oil over medium heat. Add carrot, celery, and onion, and sauté until softened.

2. Add garlic and cook for another minute.

3. Stir in lentils, diced tomatoes, vegetable broth, cumin, turmeric, and paprika. Bring to a boil.

4. Reduce heat and simmer for 25-30 minutes until lentils are tender.

5. Season with salt and pepper to taste.

6. Serve hot, garnished with fresh spinach.

Nutritional Facts (per serving):

- Calories: 250 kcal

- Protein: 13g

- Carbohydrates: 37g

- Fat: 7g

- Fiber: 13g

Mediterranean Stuffed Peppers

- **Prep Time:** 15 minutes

- **Cook Time:** 30 minutes

- **Serving Size:** 4 servings

Ingredients:

- 4 bell peppers, halved and seeded

- 1 cup cooked quinoa

- 1 cup cherry tomatoes, halved

- 1/2 cup Kalamata olives, sliced

- 1/4 cup red onion, finely chopped

- 1/2 cup feta cheese, crumbled

- 1 tablespoon olive oil

- 1 teaspoon dried oregano

- Salt and pepper to taste

Instructions:

1. Preheat oven to 375°F (190°C).

2. In a large bowl, combine cooked quinoa, cherry tomatoes, olives, red onion, feta cheese, olive oil, oregano, salt, and pepper.

3. Fill each bell pepper half with the quinoa mixture.

4. Place stuffed peppers in a baking dish and cover with foil.

5. Bake for 30 minutes until peppers are tender.

6. Serve warm.

Nutritional Facts (per serving):

- Calories: 220 kcal
- Protein: 8g
- Carbohydrates: 28g
- Fat: 10g
- Fiber: 6g

Turmeric Chicken and Rice

- **Prep Time:** 10 minutes
- **Cook Time:** 30 minutes
- **Serving Size:** 4 servings

Ingredients:

- 2 chicken breasts, diced
- 1 cup brown rice
- 2 cups water
- 1 onion, diced
- 2 garlic cloves, minced
- 1 tablespoon turmeric powder
- 1 teaspoon cumin
- 1 teaspoon paprika
- Salt and pepper to taste
- 2 tablespoons olive oil
- Fresh cilantro for garnish

Instructions:

1. In a medium pot, bring brown rice and water to a boil. Reduce heat, cover, and simmer for 30 minutes or until rice is cooked.

2. In a large skillet, heat olive oil over medium heat. Add diced chicken and cook until browned and cooked through.

3. Remove chicken from skillet and set aside.

4. In the same skillet, add onion and sauté until softened. Add garlic and cook for another minute.

5. Stir in turmeric, cumin, paprika, salt, and pepper.

6. Add cooked rice and chicken back to the skillet, stirring to combine and heat through.

7. Serve warm, garnished with fresh cilantro.

Nutritional Facts (per serving):

- Calories: 350 kcal

- Protein: 25g

- Carbohydrates: 40g

- Fat: 10g

- Fiber: 4g

Kale and Sweet Potato Salad

- **Prep Time:** 15 minutes

- **Cook Time:** 20 minutes

- **Serving Size:** 4 servings

Ingredients:

- 2 large sweet potatoes, peeled and cubed

- 1 bunch kale, stems removed and chopped

- 1/4 cup red onion, thinly sliced

- 1/4 cup dried cranberries

- 1/4 cup walnuts, chopped

- 1/4 cup feta cheese, crumbled

- 2 tablespoons olive oil

- 1 tablespoon balsamic vinegar

- Salt and pepper to taste

Instructions:

1. Preheat oven to 400°F (200°C).

2. Toss sweet potato cubes with 1 tablespoon olive oil, salt, and pepper. Spread on a baking sheet and roast for 20 minutes until tender.

3. In a large bowl, combine chopped kale, red onion, dried cranberries, walnuts, and roasted sweet potatoes.

4. In a small bowl, whisk together remaining olive oil, balsamic vinegar, salt, and pepper.

5. Pour the dressing over the salad and toss to combine.

6. Sprinkle with feta cheese before serving.

Nutritional Facts (per serving):

- Calories: 300 kcal

- Protein: 6g

- Carbohydrates: 40g

- Fat: 15g

- Fiber: 7g

Salmon and Avocado Wrap

- **Prep Time:** 10 minutes
- **Cook Time:** 10 minutes
- **Serving Size:** 2 servings

Ingredients:

- 2 whole-grain tortillas
- 1 cup cooked salmon, flaked
- 1 avocado, sliced
- 1/2 cup cherry tomatoes, halved
- 1/4 cup red onion, thinly sliced
- 1/4 cup fresh spinach
- 2 tablespoons hummus
- Salt and pepper to taste

Instructions:

1. Spread 1 tablespoon of hummus on each tortilla.
2. Layer with fresh spinach, flaked salmon, avocado slices, cherry tomatoes, and red onion.
3. Season with salt and pepper.
4. Roll up the tortillas, cut in half, and serve immediately.

Nutritional Facts (per serving):

- Calories: 350 kcal
- Protein: 22g
- Carbohydrates: 30g

- Fat: 18g

- Fiber: 8g

Chickpea and Spinach Curry

- **Prep Time:** 10 minutes

- **Cook Time:** 20 minutes

- **Serving Size:** 4 servings

Ingredients:

- 1 can (15 oz) chickpeas, drained and rinsed

- 4 cups fresh spinach

- 1 onion, diced

- 2 garlic cloves, minced

- 1 can (14.5 oz) diced tomatoes

- 1 cup coconut milk

- 1 tablespoon curry powder

- 1 teaspoon turmeric

- Salt and pepper to taste

- 2 tablespoons olive oil

- Fresh cilantro for garnish

Instructions:

1. In a large skillet, heat olive oil over medium heat. Add onion and sauté until softened.

2. Add garlic and cook for another minute.

3. Stir in curry powder and turmeric, cooking for 1-2 minutes until fragrant.

4. Add chickpeas, diced tomatoes, and coconut milk. Bring to a simmer.

5. Stir in fresh spinach and cook until wilted.

6. Season with salt and pepper.

7. Serve warm, garnished with fresh cilantro.

Nutritional Facts (per serving):

- Calories: 290 kcal

- Protein: 9g

- Carbohydrates: 30g

- Fat: 16g

- Fiber: 7g

Zucchini Noodles with Pesto

- **Prep Time:** 10 minutes

- **Cook Time:** 5 minutes

- **Serving Size:** 2 servings

Ingredients:

- 2 large zucchinis, spiralized

- 1 cup cherry tomatoes, halved

- 1/4 cup fresh basil leaves

- 1/4 cup pine nuts

- 1/4 cup grated Parmesan cheese

- 1 garlic clove

- 2 tablespoons olive oil

- Salt and pepper to taste

Instructions:

1. In a blender or food processor, combine basil leaves, pine nuts, grated Parmesan cheese, garlic, olive oil, salt, and pepper. Blend until smooth to make pesto.

2. In a large skillet, heat 1 tablespoon olive oil over medium heat. Add zucchini noodles and sauté for 2-3 minutes until just tender.

3. Add cherry tomatoes and cook for another 2 minutes.

4. Remove from heat and toss with prepared pesto.

5. Serve immediately.

Nutritional Facts (per serving):

- Calories: 250 kcal

- Protein: 8g

- Carbohydrates: 12g

- Fat: 20g

- Fiber: 4g

Black Bean and Corn Tacos

- **Prep Time:** 10 minutes

- **Cook Time:** 10 minutes

- **Serving Size:** 4 servings

Ingredients:

- 8 small corn tortillas

- 1 can (15 oz) black beans, drained and rinsed

- 1 cup corn kernels (fresh or frozen)

- 1/2 cup red onion, diced

- 1 avocado, diced

- 1/4 cup fresh cilantro, chopped

- 1 lime, cut into wedges

- 1 teaspoon cumin

- 1 teaspoon chili powder

- Salt and pepper to taste

- 2 tablespoons olive oil

Instructions:

1. In a large skillet, heat olive oil over medium heat. Add red onion and sauté until softened.

2. Stir in black beans, corn, cumin, and chili powder. Cook until heated through.

3. Season with salt and pepper.

4. Warm corn tortillas in a separate skillet or microwave.

5. Fill tortillas with black bean and corn mixture.

6. Top with diced avocado and fresh cilantro. Serve with lime wedges.

Nutritional Facts (per serving):

- Calories: 300 kcal

- Protein: 10g

- Carbohydrates: 45g

- Fat: 10g

- Fiber: 10g

Baked Falafel with Tzatziki

- **Prep Time:** 15 minutes

- **Cook Time:** 20 minutes

- **Serving Size:** 4 servings

Ingredients:

- 1 can (15 oz) chickpeas, drained and rinsed

- 1/2 onion, chopped

- 2 garlic cloves

- 1/4 cup fresh parsley

- 1 teaspoon cumin

- 1 teaspoon coriander

- Salt and pepper to taste

- 2 tablespoons olive oil

- 1 cup Greek yogurt

- 1/2 cucumber, grated

- 1 tablespoon fresh dill, chopped

- 1 tablespoon lemon juice

- 1 garlic clove, minced

Instructions:

1. Preheat oven to 375°F (190°C) and grease a baking sheet with olive oil.

2. In a food processor, combine chickpeas, onion, garlic, parsley, cumin, coriander, salt, and pepper. Pulse until well combined but not smooth.

3. Form mixture into small patties and place on the prepared baking sheet.

4. Brush the falafel patties with olive oil and bake for 20 minutes, flipping halfway through.

5. While falafel is baking, make the tzatziki sauce by combining Greek yogurt, grated cucumber, fresh dill, lemon juice, and minced garlic in a bowl. Mix well.

6. Serve baked falafel with tzatziki sauce.

Nutritional Facts (per serving):

- Calories: 280 kcal

- Protein: 12g

- Carbohydrates: 30g

- Fat: 12g

- Fiber: 8g

Spinach and Feta Stuffed Chicken Breast

- **Prep Time:** 10 minutes

- **Cook Time:** 25 minutes

- **Serving Size:** 2 servings

Ingredients:

- 2 boneless, skinless chicken breasts

- 1 cup fresh spinach, chopped

- 1/4 cup feta cheese, crumbled

- 1 garlic clove, minced

- 1 tablespoon olive oil

- Salt and pepper to taste

Instructions:

1. Preheat oven to 375°F (190°C).

2. In a bowl, mix together chopped spinach, feta cheese, and minced garlic.

3. Cut a pocket in each chicken breast and stuff with the spinach mixture.

4. Secure with toothpicks if needed.

5. Season the outside of the chicken breasts with salt and pepper.

6. Heat olive oil in an oven-safe skillet over medium heat. Sear chicken breasts for 2-3 minutes on each side until browned.

7. Transfer the skillet to the oven and bake for 20 minutes until the chicken is cooked through.

8. Remove toothpicks before serving.

Nutritional Facts (per serving):

- Calories: 300 kcal

- Protein: 35g

- Carbohydrates: 2g

- Fat: 16g

- Fiber: 1g

Roasted Veggie Buddha Bowl

- **Prep Time:** 15 minutes

- **Cook Time:** 25 minutes

- **Serving Size:** 4 servings

Ingredients:

- 2 cups cooked brown rice

- 1 cup broccoli florets

- 1 cup cauliflower florets

- 1 red bell pepper, diced

- 1 zucchini, sliced

- 1 tablespoon olive oil

- Salt and pepper to taste

- 1 avocado, sliced

- 1/4 cup tahini

- 2 tablespoons lemon juice

- 1 garlic clove, minced

- Water to thin

Instructions:

1. Preheat oven to 400°F (200°C).

2. Toss broccoli, cauliflower, red bell pepper, and zucchini with olive oil, salt, and pepper. Spread on a baking sheet.

3. Roast for 20-25 minutes until vegetables are tender and slightly browned.

4. In a small bowl, whisk together tahini, lemon juice, minced garlic, and water to desired consistency.

5. In bowls, divide cooked brown rice and top with roasted vegetables and sliced avocado.

6. Drizzle with tahini sauce before serving.

Nutritional Facts (per serving):

- Calories: 350 kcal

- Protein: 10g

- Carbohydrates: 50g

- Fat: 15g

- Fiber: 10g

Sweet Potato and Black Bean Burrito Bowl

- **Prep Time:** 15 minutes

- **Cook Time:** 20 minutes

- **Serving Size:** 4 servings

Ingredients:

- 2 large sweet potatoes, peeled and cubed

- 1 can (15 oz) black beans, drained and rinsed

- 1 cup cooked brown rice

- 1 cup corn kernels (fresh or frozen)
- 1 avocado, diced
- 1/4 cup red onion, diced
- 1/4 cup fresh cilantro, chopped
- 1 lime, cut into wedges
- 1 teaspoon cumin
- 1 teaspoon paprika
- Salt and pepper to taste
- 2 tablespoons olive oil

Instructions:

1. Preheat oven to 400°F (200°C).

2. Toss sweet potato cubes with 1 tablespoon olive oil, cumin, paprika, salt, and pepper. Spread on a baking sheet and roast for 20 minutes until tender.

3. In a large bowl, combine cooked brown rice, black beans, corn, diced avocado, red onion, and roasted sweet potatoes.

4. Drizzle with remaining olive oil and toss gently.

5. Garnish with fresh cilantro and serve with lime wedges.

Nutritional Facts (per serving):

- Calories: 400 kcal
- Protein: 12g
- Carbohydrates: 65g
- Fat: 13g
- Fiber: 15g

Greek Quinoa Salad

- **Prep Time:** 15 minutes

- **Cook Time:** 15 minutes

- **Serving Size:** 4 servings

Ingredients:

- 1 cup quinoa, rinsed

- 2 cups water

- 1 cup cherry tomatoes, halved

- 1 cucumber, diced

- 1/2 cup Kalamata olives, sliced

- 1/4 cup red onion, finely chopped

- 1/2 cup feta cheese, crumbled

- 1/4 cup fresh parsley, chopped

- 1/4 cup olive oil

- 2 tablespoons red wine vinegar

- 1 garlic clove, minced

- Salt and pepper to taste

Instructions:

1. In a medium pot, bring quinoa and water to a boil. Reduce heat, cover, and simmer for 15 minutes until quinoa is cooked. Let cool.

2. In a large bowl, combine cooked quinoa, cherry tomatoes, cucumber, olives, red onion, feta cheese, and parsley.

3. In a small bowl, whisk together olive oil, red wine vinegar, minced garlic, salt, and pepper.

4. Pour the dressing over the salad and toss to combine.

5. Serve immediately or refrigerate for later.

Nutritional Facts (per serving):

- Calories: 320 kcal

- Protein: 10g

- Carbohydrates: 32g

- Fat: 18g

- Fiber: 5g

Thai Peanut Chicken Salad

- **Prep Time:** 15 minutes

- **Cook Time:** 10 minutes

- **Serving Size:** 4 servings

Ingredients:

- 2 cups cooked chicken breast, shredded

- 2 cups shredded cabbage

- 1 cup shredded carrots

- 1 red bell pepper, thinly sliced

- 1/4 cup fresh cilantro, chopped

- 1/4 cup green onions, sliced

- 1/4 cup peanuts, chopped

- 1/4 cup peanut butter

- 2 tablespoons soy sauce (or tamari for gluten-free)

- 1 tablespoon rice vinegar

- 1 tablespoon honey or maple syrup

- 1 teaspoon sesame oil

- 1 garlic clove, minced

- 1 tablespoon lime juice

Instructions:

1. In a large bowl, combine shredded chicken, cabbage, carrots, red bell pepper, cilantro, and green onions.

2. In a small bowl, whisk together peanut butter, soy sauce, rice vinegar, honey or maple syrup, sesame oil, minced garlic, and lime juice until smooth.

3. Pour the dressing over the salad and toss to combine.

4. Garnish with chopped peanuts before serving.

Nutritional Facts (per serving):

- Calories: 350 kcal

- Protein: 25g

- Carbohydrates: 20g

- Fat: 18g

- Fiber: 5g

Chapter 5: Dinner Recipes

Blueberry Chia Seed Pudding

- **Prep Time:** 10 minutes

- **Cook Time:** 0 minutes (refrigerate overnight)

- **Serving Size:** 2 servings

Ingredients:

- 1 cup unsweetened almond milk

- 1/4 cup chia seeds

- 1 cup blueberries

- 1 tablespoon maple syrup

- 1/2 teaspoon vanilla extract

Instructions:

1. In a bowl, combine almond milk, chia seeds, blueberries, maple syrup, and vanilla extract.

2. Stir well and refrigerate overnight.

3. In the morning, stir again and serve chilled.

Nutritional Facts (per serving):

- Calories: 190 kcal

- Protein: 5g

- Carbohydrates: 28g

- Fat: 8g

- Fiber: 12g

Avocado Toast with Smoked Salmon

- **Prep Time:** 10 minutes

- **Cook Time:** 5 minutes

- **Serving Size:** 2 servings

Ingredients:

- 2 slices whole-grain bread

- 1 ripe avocado

- 4 oz smoked salmon

- 1 tablespoon lemon juice

- Salt and pepper to taste

- Red pepper flakes (optional)

Instructions:

1. Toast the bread slices to your preference.

2. Mash the avocado in a bowl and mix with lemon juice, salt, and pepper.

3. Spread the avocado mixture on the toast.

4. Top with smoked salmon and sprinkle with red pepper flakes if desired.

Nutritional Facts (per serving):

- Calories: 250 kcal

- Protein: 12g

- Carbohydrates: 22g

- Fat: 15g

- Fiber: 7g

Turmeric Oatmeal

- **Prep Time:** 5 minutes

- **Cook Time:** 10 minutes

- **Serving Size:** 2 servings

Ingredients:

- 1 cup rolled oats

- 2 cups water or unsweetened almond milk

- 1/2 teaspoon ground turmeric

- 1/4 teaspoon ground cinnamon

- 1 tablespoon honey or maple syrup

- Fresh fruit for topping (e.g., berries, banana slices)

Instructions:

1. In a saucepan, bring water or almond milk to a boil.

2. Add oats, turmeric, and cinnamon, reduce heat, and simmer for 5-7 minutes, stirring occasionally.

3. Stir in honey or maple syrup.

4. Serve topped with fresh fruit.

Nutritional Facts (per serving):

- Calories: 220 kcal

- Protein: 6g

- Carbohydrates: 38g

- Fat: 4g

- Fiber: 6g

Green Smoothie Bowl

- **Prep Time:** 10 minutes
- **Cook Time:** 0 minutes
- **Serving Size:** 2 servings

Ingredients:

- 2 cups spinach
- 1 frozen banana
- 1/2 avocado
- 1 cup unsweetened almond milk
- 1 tablespoon chia seeds
- Fresh fruit and nuts for topping

Instructions:

1. Blend spinach, banana, avocado, and almond milk until smooth.
2. Pour into bowls and top with chia seeds, fresh fruit, and nuts.

Nutritional Facts (per serving):

- Calories: 250 kcal
- Protein: 4g
- Carbohydrates: 28g
- Fat: 14g
- Fiber: 9g

Sweet Potato Breakfast Hash

- **Prep Time:** 10 minutes

- **Cook Time:** 20 minutes

- **Serving Size:** 2 servings

Ingredients:

- 2 medium sweet potatoes, peeled and diced

- 1 red bell pepper, diced

- 1 small onion, diced

- 2 tablespoons olive oil

- 1 teaspoon smoked paprika

- Salt and pepper to taste

- 2 eggs (optional)

Instructions:

1. In a large skillet, heat olive oil over medium heat.

2. Add sweet potatoes, bell pepper, and onion. Season with smoked paprika, salt, and pepper.

3. Cook, stirring occasionally, until sweet potatoes are tender, about 15-20 minutes.

4. If desired, fry or poach eggs separately and serve on top of the hash.

Nutritional Facts (per serving, without eggs):

- Calories: 250 kcal
- Protein: 3g
- Carbohydrates: 40g
- Fat: 10g

- Fiber: 6g

Quinoa Breakfast Bowl

- **Prep Time:** 5 minutes

- **Cook Time:** 15 minutes

- **Serving Size:** 2 servings

Ingredients:

- 1 cup cooked quinoa

- 1 cup almond milk

- 1 banana, sliced

- 1 tablespoon almond butter

- 1 tablespoon chia seeds

- 1 tablespoon honey or maple syrup

Instructions:

1. In a saucepan, combine cooked quinoa and almond milk. Heat over medium heat until warm.

2. Divide between bowls and top with banana slices, almond butter, chia seeds, and honey or maple syrup.

Nutritional Facts (per serving):

- Calories: 300 kcal

- Protein: 8g

- Carbohydrates: 50g

- Fat: 10g

- Fiber: 6g

Apple Cinnamon Overnight Oats

- **Prep Time:** 10 minutes

- **Cook Time:** 0 minutes (refrigerate overnight)

- **Serving Size:** 2 servings

Ingredients:

- 1 cup rolled oats

- 1 cup unsweetened almond milk

- 1 apple, grated

- 1 teaspoon ground cinnamon

- 1 tablespoon chia seeds

- 1 tablespoon honey or maple syrup

Instructions:

1. In a bowl, combine rolled oats, almond milk, grated apple, cinnamon, chia seeds, and honey or maple syrup.

2. Stir well and refrigerate overnight.

3. In the morning, stir again and serve chilled.

Nutritional Facts (per serving):

- Calories: 220 kcal

- Protein: 5g

- Carbohydrates: 45g

- Fat: 4g

- Fiber: 7g

Spinach and Mushroom Omelette

- **Prep Time:** 5 minutes

- **Cook Time:** 10 minutes

- **Serving Size:** 1 serving

Ingredients:

- 2 eggs

- 1/2 cup spinach, chopped

- 1/4 cup mushrooms, sliced

- 1 tablespoon olive oil

- Salt and pepper to taste

Instructions:

1. In a bowl, whisk eggs with salt and pepper.

2. Heat olive oil in a skillet over medium heat. Add mushrooms and cook until softened.

3. Add spinach and cook until wilted.

4. Pour in eggs and cook until set, folding the omelette in half.

5. Serve warm.

Nutritional Facts (per serving):

- Calories: 200 kcal

- Protein: 12g

- Carbohydrates: 3g

- Fat: 16g

- Fiber: 1g

Berry Smoothie

- **Prep Time:** 5 minutes

- **Cook Time:** 0 minutes

- **Serving Size:** 2 servings

Ingredients:

- 1 cup mixed berries (fresh or frozen)

- 1 banana

- 1 cup unsweetened almond milk

- 1 tablespoon chia seeds

- 1 tablespoon honey or maple syrup (optional)

Instructions:

1. Combine all ingredients in a blender and blend until smooth.

2. Pour into glasses and serve immediately.

Nutritional Facts (per serving):

- Calories: 150 kcal

- Protein: 2g

- Carbohydrates: 33g

- Fat: 4g

- Fiber: 7g

Almond Butter and Banana Toast

- **Prep Time:** 5 minutes

- **Cook Time:** 5 minutes

- **Serving Size:** 2 servings

Ingredients:

- 2 slices whole-grain bread

- 2 tablespoons almond butter

- 1 banana, sliced

- 1 teaspoon chia seeds

- Cinnamon for sprinkling

Instructions:

1. Toast the bread slices.

2. Spread almond butter on each slice.

3. Top with banana slices and sprinkle with chia seeds and cinnamon.

Nutritional Facts (per serving):

- Calories: 250 kcal

- Protein: 7g

- Carbohydrates: 35g

- Fat: 10g

- Fiber: 6g

Turmeric Smoothie

- **Prep Time:** 5 minutes
- **Cook Time:** 0 minutes
- **Serving Size:** 2 servings

Ingredients:

- 1 cup unsweetened almond milk
- 1 banana
- 1/2 cup frozen pineapple chunks
- 1/2 teaspoon ground turmeric
- 1/2 teaspoon ground ginger
- 1 tablespoon chia seeds
- 1 teaspoon honey or maple syrup (optional)

Instructions:

1. Combine all ingredients in a blender.
2. Blend until smooth.
3. Pour into glasses and serve immediately.

Nutritional Facts (per serving):

- Calories: 140 kcal
- Protein: 2g
- Carbohydrates: 30g
- Fat: 3g
- Fiber: 6g

Coconut Yogurt Parfait

- **Prep Time:** 5 minutes
- **Cook Time:** 0 minutes
- **Serving Size:** 2 servings

Ingredients:

- 1 cup coconut yogurt
- 1/2 cup granola (preferably low-sugar)
- 1/2 cup mixed berries
- 1 tablespoon chia seeds
- 1 tablespoon honey or maple syrup (optional)

Instructions:

1. In two glasses, layer coconut yogurt, granola, mixed berries, and chia seeds.
2. Drizzle with honey or maple syrup if desired.
3. Serve immediately.

Nutritional Facts (per serving):

- Calories: 250 kcal
- Protein: 4g
- Carbohydrates: 35g
- Fat: 12g
- Fiber: 7g

Savory Chickpea Pancakes

- **Prep Time:** 10 minutes

- **Cook Time:** 15 minutes

- **Serving Size:** 2 servings

Ingredients:

- 1 cup chickpea flour

- 1 cup water

- 1/2 teaspoon turmeric

- 1/2 teaspoon cumin

- 1/2 cup chopped spinach

- 1/4 cup grated carrot

- 1 tablespoon olive oil

- Salt and pepper to taste

Instructions:

1. In a bowl, whisk together chickpea flour, water, turmeric, cumin, salt, and pepper until smooth.

2. Stir in chopped spinach and grated carrot.

3. Heat olive oil in a skillet over medium heat.

4. Pour batter into the skillet to form small pancakes.

5. Cook for 3-4 minutes on each side until golden brown.

6. Serve warm.

Nutritional Facts (per serving):

- Calories: 200 kcal

- Protein: 8g

- Carbohydrates: 30g

- Fat: 6g

- Fiber: 6g

Buckwheat Porridge

- **Prep Time:** 5 minutes

- **Cook Time:** 15 minutes

- **Serving Size:** 2 servings

Ingredients:

- 1 cup buckwheat groats

- 2 cups water or unsweetened almond milk

- 1 apple, diced

- 1 teaspoon ground cinnamon

- 1 tablespoon honey or maple syrup

- 1 tablespoon flaxseeds

Instructions:

1. In a pot, combine buckwheat groats and water or almond milk. Bring to a boil.

2. Reduce heat and simmer for 10-15 minutes until buckwheat is tender.

3. Stir in diced apple, cinnamon, and honey or maple syrup.

4. Serve topped with flaxseeds.

Nutritional Facts (per serving):

- Calories: 240 kcal

- Protein: 6g

- Carbohydrates: 48g

- Fat: 4g

- Fiber: 8g

Matcha Green Tea Smoothie

- **Prep Time:** 5 minutes

- **Cook Time:** 0 minutes

- **Serving Size:** 2 servings

Ingredients:

- 1 cup unsweetened almond milk

- 1 banana

- 1/2 cup spinach

- 1 teaspoon matcha green tea powder

- 1 tablespoon chia seeds

- 1 teaspoon honey or maple syrup (optional)

Instructions:

1. Combine all ingredients in a blender.

2. Blend until smooth.

3. Pour into glasses and serve immediately.

Nutritional Facts (per serving):

- Calories: 120 kcal

- Protein: 3g

- Carbohydrates: 26g

- Fat: 2g

- Fiber: 6g

Chapter 6: Snacks and Appetizers Recipes

Hummus with Veggie Sticks

- **Prep Time:** 10 minutes

- **Cook Time:** 0 minutes

- **Serving Size:** 4 servings

Ingredients:

- 1 can (15 oz) chickpeas, drained and rinsed

- 1/4 cup tahini

- 2 tablespoons olive oil

- 2 tablespoons lemon juice

- 1 garlic clove, minced

- 1/2 teaspoon cumin

- Salt and pepper to taste

- Assorted vegetable sticks (carrots, celery, bell peppers, cucumbers)

Instructions:

1. In a food processor, blend chickpeas, tahini, olive oil, lemon juice, garlic, cumin, salt, and pepper until smooth.

2. Adjust seasoning to taste.

3. Serve with assorted vegetable sticks.

Nutritional Facts (per serving):

- Calories: 180 kcal

- Protein: 6g

- Carbohydrates: 20g

- Fat: 8g

- Fiber: 6g

Turmeric Roasted Chickpeas

- **Prep Time:** 10 minutes

- **Cook Time:** 30 minutes

- **Serving Size:** 4 servings

Ingredients:

- 1 can (15 oz) chickpeas, drained and rinsed

- 1 tablespoon olive oil

- 1 teaspoon ground turmeric

- 1/2 teaspoon cumin

- 1/2 teaspoon paprika

- Salt and pepper to taste

Instructions:

1. Preheat oven to 400°F (200°C).

2. Pat chickpeas dry with a paper towel.

3. In a bowl, toss chickpeas with olive oil, turmeric, cumin, paprika, salt, and pepper.

4. Spread chickpeas on a baking sheet and roast for 30 minutes, stirring halfway through.

5. Let cool and serve.

Nutritional Facts (per serving):

- Calories: 150 kcal

- Protein: 5g

- Carbohydrates: 20g

- Fat: 5g

- Fiber: 5g

Guacamole with Flaxseed Crackers

- **Prep Time:** 10 minutes

- **Cook Time:** 0 minutes

- **Serving Size:** 4 servings

Ingredients:

- 2 ripe avocados

- 1/4 cup red onion, finely chopped

- 1 small tomato, diced

- 1 tablespoon lime juice

- 1 garlic clove, minced

- Salt and pepper to taste

- Flaxseed crackers

Instructions:

1. In a bowl, mash avocados with a fork.

2. Stir in red onion, tomato, lime juice, garlic, salt, and pepper.

3. Serve with flaxseed crackers.

Nutritional Facts (per serving):

- Calories: 200 kcal

- Protein: 3g

- Carbohydrates: 12g

- Fat: 18g

- Fiber: 8g

Baked Sweet Potato Fries

- **Prep Time:** 10 minutes

- **Cook Time:** 25 minutes

- **Serving Size:** 4 servings

Ingredients:

- 2 large sweet potatoes, peeled and cut into fries

- 2 tablespoons olive oil

- 1 teaspoon paprika

- 1/2 teaspoon garlic powder

- Salt and pepper to taste

Instructions:

1. Preheat oven to 425°F (220°C).

2. In a bowl, toss sweet potato fries with olive oil, paprika, garlic powder, salt, and pepper.

3. Spread fries on a baking sheet in a single layer.

4. Bake for 25 minutes, flipping halfway through, until crispy.

5. Serve immediately.

Nutritional Facts (per serving):

- Calories: 180 kcal

- Protein: 2g

- Carbohydrates: 30g

- Fat: 6g

- Fiber: 5g

Stuffed Mini Bell Peppers

- **Prep Time:** 15 minutes

- **Cook Time:** 0 minutes

- **Serving Size:** 4 servings

Ingredients:

- 12 mini bell peppers

- 1 cup hummus

- 1/4 cup chopped fresh parsley

- 1 tablespoon lemon juice

- Salt and pepper to taste

Instructions:

1. Slice the tops off mini bell peppers and remove seeds.

2. In a bowl, mix hummus with parsley, lemon juice, salt, and pepper.

3. Fill each bell pepper with the hummus mixture.

4. Serve chilled.

Nutritional Facts (per serving):

- Calories: 100 kcal

- Protein: 3g

- Carbohydrates: 12g

- Fat: 5g

- Fiber: 4g

Chia Seed Pudding

- **Prep Time:** 5 minutes

- **Cook Time:** 0 minutes (refrigerate overnight)

- **Serving Size:** 4 servings

Ingredients:

- 2 cups unsweetened almond milk

- 1/2 cup chia seeds

- 2 tablespoons maple syrup

- 1 teaspoon vanilla extract

- Fresh fruit for topping

Instructions:

1. In a bowl, combine almond milk, chia seeds, maple syrup, and vanilla extract.

2. Stir well and refrigerate overnight.

3. In the morning, stir again and top with fresh fruit.

4. Serve chilled.

Nutritional Facts (per serving):

- Calories: 150 kcal

- Protein: 4g

- Carbohydrates: 15g

- Fat: 8g

- Fiber: 8g

Kale Chips

- **Prep Time:** 10 minutes

- **Cook Time:** 20 minutes

- **Serving Size:** 4 servings

Ingredients:

- 1 bunch kale, stems removed and leaves torn into bite-sized pieces

- 1 tablespoon olive oil

- 1/2 teaspoon sea salt

Instructions:

1. Preheat oven to 300°F (150°C).

2. In a bowl, toss kale leaves with olive oil and sea salt.

3. Spread kale in a single layer on a baking sheet.

4. Bake for 20 minutes, until crisp.

5. Serve immediately.

Nutritional Facts (per serving):

- Calories: 50 kcal

- Protein: 2g

- Carbohydrates: 7g

- Fat: 2g

- Fiber: 2g

Almond Butter Energy Bites

- **Prep Time:** 15 minutes

- **Cook Time:** 0 minutes

- **Serving Size:** 12 bites

Ingredients:

- 1 cup rolled oats

- 1/2 cup almond butter

- 1/4 cup honey or maple syrup

- 1/4 cup chia seeds

- 1/4 cup dark chocolate chips

Instructions:

1. In a bowl, mix together rolled oats, almond butter, honey or maple syrup, chia seeds, and dark chocolate chips.

2. Roll mixture into small balls and place on a baking sheet.

3. Refrigerate for at least 30 minutes before serving.

Nutritional Facts (per bite):

- Calories: 100 kcal
- Protein: 2g
- Carbohydrates: 12g
- Fat: 5g

- Fiber: 2g

Greek Yogurt with Honey and Walnuts

- **Prep Time:** 5 minutes

- **Cook Time:** 0 minutes

- **Serving Size:** 2 servings

Ingredients:

- 1 cup Greek yogurt

- 2 tablespoons honey

- 1/4 cup walnuts, chopped

- 1 teaspoon ground cinnamon

Instructions:

1. Divide Greek yogurt between two bowls.

2. Drizzle with honey.

3. Top with chopped walnuts and a sprinkle of cinnamon.

4. Serve immediately.

Nutritional Facts (per serving):

- Calories: 200 kcal

- Protein: 10g

- Carbohydrates: 20g

- Fat: 10g

- Fiber: 2g

Edamame with Sea Salt

- **Prep Time:** 5 minutes

- **Cook Time:** 5 minutes

- **Serving Size:** 4 servings

Ingredients:

- 2 cups edamame (in pods)

- 1 teaspoon sea salt

Instructions:

1. Bring a pot of water to a boil.

2. Add edamame and cook for 5 minutes, until tender.

3. Drain and sprinkle with sea salt.

4. Serve warm or cold.

Nutritional Facts (per serving):

- Calories: 90 kcal

- Protein: 8g

- Carbohydrates: 8g

- Fat: 3g

- Fiber: 4g

Chapter 7: Desserts Recipes

Berry Chia Pudding

- **Prep Time:** 10 minutes

- **Cook Time:** 0 minutes (refrigerate overnight)

- **Serving Size:** 4 servings

Ingredients:

- 2 cups unsweetened almond milk

- 1/2 cup chia seeds

- 2 tablespoons maple syrup

- 1 teaspoon vanilla extract

- 1 cup mixed berries

Instructions:

1. In a bowl, whisk together almond milk, chia seeds, maple syrup, and vanilla extract.

2. Let it sit for about 5 minutes, then whisk again to prevent clumping.

3. Cover and refrigerate overnight.

4. Before serving, stir well and top with mixed berries.

Nutritional Facts (per serving):

- Calories: 160 kcal

- Protein: 4g

- Carbohydrates: 18g

- Fat: 8g

- Fiber: 9g

Dark Chocolate Avocado Mousse

- **Prep Time:** 10 minutes
- **Cook Time:** 0 minutes
- **Serving Size:** 4 servings

Ingredients:

- 2 ripe avocados
- 1/4 cup cocoa powder
- 1/4 cup maple syrup
- 1 teaspoon vanilla extract
- Pinch of sea salt

Instructions:

1. In a blender or food processor, combine all ingredients and blend until smooth.
2. Spoon the mousse into serving dishes and refrigerate for at least 30 minutes before serving.

Nutritional Facts (per serving):

- Calories: 210 kcal
- Protein: 3g
- Carbohydrates: 29g
- Fat: 12g
- Fiber: 7g

Coconut Macaroons

- **Prep Time:** 10 minutes

- **Cook Time:** 20 minutes

- **Serving Size:** 12 macaroons

Ingredients:

- 2 cups unsweetened shredded coconut

- 1/4 cup coconut flour

- 1/4 cup maple syrup

- 1/4 cup coconut oil, melted

- 1 teaspoon vanilla extract

- Pinch of sea salt

Instructions:

1. Preheat oven to 325°F (165°C) and line a baking sheet with parchment paper.

2. In a bowl, mix all ingredients until well combined.

3. Scoop tablespoon-sized mounds onto the baking sheet.

4. Bake for 20 minutes or until golden brown.

5. Let cool before serving.

Nutritional Facts (per macaroon):

- Calories: 110 kcal
- Protein: 1g
- Carbohydrates: 7g
- Fat: 10g

- Fiber: 3g

Apple Cinnamon Baked Oatmeal Cups

- **Prep Time:** 10 minutes

- **Cook Time:** 25 minutes

- **Serving Size:** 6 cups

Ingredients:

- 2 cups rolled oats

- 1 teaspoon baking powder

- 1 teaspoon ground cinnamon

- 1/4 teaspoon sea salt

- 1 cup unsweetened applesauce

- 1 cup unsweetened almond milk

- 1 egg

- 1 apple, diced

Instructions:

1. Preheat oven to 350°F (175°C) and grease a muffin tin.

2. In a bowl, mix oats, baking powder, cinnamon, and salt.

3. In another bowl, whisk together applesauce, almond milk, and egg.

4. Combine wet and dry ingredients, then fold in diced apple.

5. Pour the mixture into the muffin tin.

6. Bake for 25 minutes or until set.

7. Let cool before serving.

Nutritional Facts (per cup):

- Calories: 110 kcal

- Protein: 3g

- Carbohydrates: 20g

- Fat: 2g

- Fiber: 3g

Mango Coconut Popsicles

- **Prep Time:** 10 minutes

- **Cook Time:** 0 minutes (freeze for 4 hours)

- **Serving Size:** 6 popsicles

Ingredients:

- 2 cups mango chunks (fresh or frozen)

- 1 cup coconut milk

- 1 tablespoon honey or maple syrup (optional)

Instructions:

1. Blend mango chunks, coconut milk, and honey or maple syrup (if using) until smooth.

2. Pour the mixture into popsicle molds.

3. Freeze for at least 4 hours or until solid.

4. To serve, run the molds under warm water to release the popsicles.

Nutritional Facts (per popsicle):

- Calories: 80 kcal

- Protein: 1g

- Carbohydrates: 15g

- Fat: 3g

- Fiber: 1g

Banana Almond Nice Cream

- **Prep Time:** 10 minutes

- **Cook Time:** 0 minutes

- **Serving Size:** 2 servings

Ingredients:

- 3 ripe bananas, sliced and frozen

- 1/4 cup almond butter

- 1 teaspoon vanilla extract

Instructions:

1. In a food processor, blend frozen banana slices, almond butter, and vanilla extract until smooth.

2. Serve immediately as soft-serve or freeze for 1-2 hours for a firmer texture.

Nutritional Facts (per serving):

- Calories: 200 kcal

- Protein: 4g

- Carbohydrates: 35g

- Fat: 7g

- Fiber: 5g

Turmeric Golden Milk Latte

- **Prep Time:** 5 minutes

- **Cook Time:** 5 minutes

- **Serving Size:** 2 servings

Ingredients:

- 2 cups unsweetened almond milk

- 1 teaspoon ground turmeric

- 1/2 teaspoon ground cinnamon

- 1/2 teaspoon ground ginger

- 1 tablespoon honey or maple syrup

- Pinch of black pepper

Instructions:

1. In a saucepan, combine all ingredients and heat over medium heat.

2. Whisk continuously until warm and well combined.

3. Pour into mugs and serve immediately.

Nutritional Facts (per serving):

- Calories: 70 kcal

- Protein: 1g

- Carbohydrates: 11g

- Fat: 3g

- Fiber: 1g

Blueberry Oat Bars

- **Prep Time:** 15 minutes

- **Cook Time:** 30 minutes

- **Serving Size:** 8 bars

Ingredients:

- 2 cups rolled oats

- 1 cup almond flour

- 1/2 cup coconut oil, melted

- 1/4 cup maple syrup

- 1 teaspoon vanilla extract

- 1 1/2 cups fresh blueberries

Instructions:

1. Preheat oven to 350°F (175°C) and line an 8x8 inch baking dish with parchment paper.

2. In a bowl, mix oats, almond flour, coconut oil, maple syrup, and vanilla extract.

3. Press half of the mixture into the bottom of the baking dish.

4. Spread blueberries evenly over the crust.

5. Crumble the remaining oat mixture on top.

6. Bake for 30 minutes or until golden brown.

7. Let cool before cutting into bars.

Nutritional Facts (per bar):

- Calories: 220 kcal

- Protein: 4g

- Carbohydrates: 24g

- Fat: 12g

- Fiber: 4g

Pumpkin Spice Energy Balls

- **Prep Time:** 15 minutes

- **Cook Time:** 0 minutes

- **Serving Size:** 12 balls

Ingredients:

- 1 cup rolled oats

- 1/2 cup pumpkin puree

- 1/4 cup almond butter

- 1/4 cup honey or maple syrup

- 1/2 teaspoon ground cinnamon

- 1/4 teaspoon ground nutmeg

- 1/4 teaspoon ground ginger

Instructions:

1. In a bowl, mix all ingredients until well combined.

2. Roll mixture into small balls and place on a baking sheet.

3. Refrigerate for at least 30 minutes before serving.

Nutritional Facts (per ball):

- Calories: 90 kcal

- Protein: 2g

- Carbohydrates: 13g

- Fat: 4g

- Fiber: 2g

Baked Pears with Walnuts and Cinnamon

- **Prep Time:** 10 minutes

- **Cook Time:** 25 minutes

- **Serving Size:** 4 servings

Ingredients:

- 2 large pears, halved and cored

- 1/4 cup walnuts, chopped

- 1 tablespoon honey or maple syrup

- 1 teaspoon ground cinnamon

Instructions:

1. Preheat oven to 350°F (175°C).
2. Place pear halves in a baking dish.
3. In a bowl, mix chopped walnuts, honey or maple syrup, and cinnamon.
4. Spoon the mixture into the pear halves.
5. Bake for 25 minutes or until pears are tender.
6. Let cool slightly before serving.

Nutritional Facts (per serving):

- Calories: 130 kcal
- Protein: 1g
- Carbohydrates: 22g
- Fat: 5g

- Fiber: 4g

Chapter 8: Beverages Recipes

Turmeric Ginger Tea

- **Prep Time:** 5 minutes

- **Cook Time:** 10 minutes

- **Serving Size:** 2 servings

Ingredients:

- 2 cups water

- 1 teaspoon ground turmeric

- 1 teaspoon grated fresh ginger

- 1 tablespoon honey or maple syrup (optional)

- Juice of 1 lemon

Instructions:

1. In a small saucepan, bring water to a boil.

2. Add turmeric and grated ginger, reduce heat and simmer for 10 minutes.

3. Strain the tea into mugs.

4. Stir in honey or maple syrup if using and add lemon juice.

5. Serve warm.

Nutritional Facts (per serving):

- Calories: 25 kcal

- Protein: 0g

- Carbohydrates: 6g

- Fat: 0g

- Fiber: 0g

Green Detox Smoothie

- **Prep Time:** 5 minutes

- **Cook Time:** 0 minutes

- **Serving Size:** 2 servings

Ingredients:

- 1 cup spinach

- 1 cup kale

- 1 green apple, cored and chopped

- 1 banana

- 1/2 cucumber

- 1 tablespoon chia seeds

- 1 cup water or coconut water

Instructions:

1. Combine all ingredients in a blender.

2. Blend until smooth.

3. Pour into glasses and serve immediately.

Nutritional Facts (per serving):

- Calories: 110 kcal

- Protein: 3g

- Carbohydrates: 25g

- Fat: 2g

- Fiber: 7g

Berry Antioxidant Smoothie

- **Prep Time:** 5 minutes

- **Cook Time:** 0 minutes

- **Serving Size:** 2 servings

Ingredients:

- 1 cup mixed berries (blueberries, raspberries, strawberries)

- 1 banana

- 1/2 cup Greek yogurt

- 1 cup unsweetened almond milk

- 1 tablespoon honey or maple syrup (optional)

Instructions:

1. Combine all ingredients in a blender.

2. Blend until smooth.

3. Pour into glasses and serve immediately.

Nutritional Facts (per serving):

- Calories: 150 kcal

- Protein: 5g

- Carbohydrates: 28g

- Fat: 3g

- Fiber: 4g

Golden Milk Latte

- **Prep Time:** 5 minutes

- **Cook Time:** 5 minutes

- **Serving Size:** 2 servings

Ingredients:

- 2 cups unsweetened almond milk

- 1 teaspoon ground turmeric

- 1/2 teaspoon ground cinnamon

- 1/2 teaspoon ground ginger

- 1 tablespoon honey or maple syrup

- Pinch of black pepper

Instructions:

1. In a saucepan, combine almond milk, turmeric, cinnamon, ginger, honey or maple syrup, and black pepper.

2. Heat over medium heat, whisking continuously until warm.

3. Pour into mugs and serve immediately.

Nutritional Facts (per serving):

- Calories: 90 kcal

- Protein: 1g

- Carbohydrates: 14g

- Fat: 3g

- Fiber: 1g

Lemon Ginger Detox Water

- **Prep Time:** 5 minutes

- **Cook Time:** 0 minutes

- **Serving Size:** 2 servings

Ingredients:

- 4 cups water

- 1 lemon, thinly sliced

- 1-inch piece fresh ginger, sliced

- Fresh mint leaves (optional)

Instructions:

1. In a pitcher, combine water, lemon slices, and ginger slices.

2. Refrigerate for at least 1 hour before serving.

3. Add fresh mint leaves if desired.

4. Serve chilled.

Nutritional Facts (per serving):

- Calories: 5 kcal

- Protein: 0g

- Carbohydrates: 1g

- Fat: 0g

- Fiber: 0g

Pineapple Turmeric Smoothie

- **Prep Time:** 5 minutes

- **Cook Time:** 0 minutes

- **Serving Size:** 2 servings

Ingredients:

- 1 cup pineapple chunks (fresh or frozen)

- 1 banana

- 1/2 teaspoon ground turmeric

- 1 cup coconut water

- 1 tablespoon chia seeds

Instructions:

1. Combine all ingredients in a blender.

2. Blend until smooth.

3. Pour into glasses and serve immediately.

Nutritional Facts (per serving):

- Calories: 120 kcal

- Protein: 2g

- Carbohydrates: 29g

- Fat: 1g

- Fiber: 5g

Matcha Green Tea Latte

- **Prep Time:** 5 minutes

- **Cook Time:** 5 minutes

- **Serving Size:** 2 servings

Ingredients:

- 2 teaspoons matcha green tea powder

- 1/4 cup hot water

- 2 cups unsweetened almond milk

- 1 tablespoon honey or maple syrup

Instructions:

1. In a small bowl, whisk matcha green tea powder with hot water until smooth.

2. In a saucepan, heat almond milk until warm.

3. Stir in honey or maple syrup.

4. Pour matcha mixture into the almond milk and whisk until frothy.

5. Pour into mugs and serve immediately.

Nutritional Facts (per serving):

- Calories: 70 kcal

- Protein: 1g

- Carbohydrates: 14g

- Fat: 2g

- Fiber: 1g

Beetroot and Berry Smoothie

- **Prep Time:** 5 minutes

- **Cook Time:** 0 minutes

- **Serving Size:** 2 servings

Ingredients:

- 1 small beet, peeled and chopped

- 1 cup mixed berries (fresh or frozen)

- 1 banana

- 1 cup unsweetened almond milk

- 1 tablespoon honey or maple syrup (optional)

Instructions:

1. Combine all ingredients in a blender.

2. Blend until smooth.

3. Pour into glasses and serve immediately.

Nutritional Facts (per serving):

- Calories: 130 kcal

- Protein: 2g

- Carbohydrates: 30g

- Fat: 2g

- Fiber: 6g

Cucumber Mint Cooler

- **Prep Time:** 5 minutes

- **Cook Time:** 0 minutes

- **Serving Size:** 2 servings

Ingredients:

- 1 cucumber, peeled and sliced

- 2 cups water

- Juice of 1 lemon

- Fresh mint leaves

- 1 tablespoon honey or maple syrup (optional)

Instructions:

1. In a blender, combine cucumber, water, lemon juice, mint leaves, and honey or maple syrup (if using).

2. Blend until smooth.

3. Strain the mixture through a fine-mesh sieve into a pitcher.

4. Serve chilled.

Nutritional Facts (per serving):

- Calories: 20 kcal

- Protein: 0g

- Carbohydrates: 5g

- Fat: 0g

- Fiber: 0g

Anti-Inflammatory Green Juice

- **Prep Time:** 5 minutes

- **Cook Time:** 0 minutes

- **Serving Size:** 2 servings

Ingredients:

- 1 cucumber

- 2 celery stalks

- 1 green apple

- 1 cup spinach

- 1-inch piece fresh ginger

- Juice of 1 lemon

Instructions:

1. In a juicer, combine cucumber, celery, green apple, spinach, and ginger.

2. Juice the ingredients and pour into glasses.

3. Stir in lemon juice.

4. Serve immediately.

Nutritional Facts (per serving):

- Calories: 50 kcal

- Protein: 1g

- Carbohydrates: 12g

- Fat: 0g

- Fiber: 2g

Chapter 9: Special Diet Considerations Recipes

Gluten-Free Quinoa Salad

- **Prep Time:** 10 minutes

- **Cook Time:** 15 minutes

- **Serving Size:** 4 servings

Ingredients:

- 1 cup quinoa, rinsed

- 2 cups water

- 1 cup cherry tomatoes, halved

- 1 cucumber, diced

- 1/4 cup red onion, finely chopped

- 1/4 cup fresh parsley, chopped

- 2 tablespoons olive oil

- 1 lemon, juiced

- Salt and pepper to taste

Instructions:

1. In a medium saucepan, bring quinoa and water to a boil. Reduce heat, cover, and simmer for 15 minutes or until water is absorbed.

2. Fluff quinoa with a fork and let it cool.

3. In a large bowl, combine cooked quinoa, cherry tomatoes, cucumber, red onion, and parsley.

4. Drizzle with olive oil and lemon juice, then season with salt and pepper.

5. Toss to combine and serve.

Nutritional Facts (per serving):

- Calories: 190 kcal

- Protein: 5g

- Carbohydrates: 28g

- Fat: 7g

- Fiber: 4g

Dairy-Free Butternut Squash Soup

- **Prep Time:** 10 minutes

- **Cook Time:** 30 minutes

- **Serving Size:** 4 servings

Ingredients:

- 1 large butternut squash, peeled and cubed

- 1 onion, chopped

- 2 garlic cloves, minced

- 4 cups vegetable broth

- 1 teaspoon ground ginger

- 1 teaspoon ground turmeric

- Salt and pepper to taste

- 1 tablespoon olive oil

Instructions:

1. Heat olive oil in a large pot over medium heat. Add onion and garlic, and sauté until translucent.

2. Add butternut squash, vegetable broth, ginger, and turmeric.

3. Bring to a boil, then reduce heat and simmer for 20 minutes, or until squash is tender.

4. Use an immersion blender to puree the soup until smooth.

5. Season with salt and pepper to taste.

6. Serve hot.

Nutritional Facts (per serving):

- Calories: 140 kcal

- Protein: 3g

- Carbohydrates: 31g

- Fat: 3g

- Fiber: 5g

Vegan Stuffed Bell Peppers

- **Prep Time:** 15 minutes

- **Cook Time:** 40 minutes

- **Serving Size:** 4 servings

Ingredients:

- 4 bell peppers, tops cut off and seeds removed

- 1 cup cooked brown rice

- 1 can black beans, drained and rinsed

- 1 cup corn kernels

- 1 onion, chopped

- 2 garlic cloves, minced

- 1 teaspoon ground cumin

- 1 teaspoon paprika

- Salt and pepper to taste

- 1 tablespoon olive oil

Instructions:

1. Preheat oven to 375°F (190°C).

2. In a large skillet, heat olive oil over medium heat. Add onion and garlic, and sauté until translucent.

3. Stir in cooked rice, black beans, corn, cumin, and paprika. Season with salt and pepper.

4. Stuff each bell pepper with the rice mixture and place in a baking dish.

5. Cover with foil and bake for 30 minutes. Remove foil and bake for an additional 10 minutes.

6. Serve warm.

Nutritional Facts (per serving):

- Calories: 250 kcal

- Protein: 8g

- Carbohydrates: 50g

- Fat: 4g

- Fiber: 10g

Low-Sugar Chia Seed Pudding

- **Prep Time:** 10 minutes

- **Cook Time:** 0 minutes (refrigerate overnight)

- **Serving Size:** 2 servings

Ingredients:

- 1 cup unsweetened almond milk

- 1/4 cup chia seeds

- 1/2 teaspoon vanilla extract

- 1 tablespoon stevia or monk fruit sweetener

- Fresh berries for topping

Instructions:

1. In a bowl, whisk together almond milk, chia seeds, vanilla extract, and sweetener.

2. Let sit for 5 minutes, then whisk again to prevent clumping.

3. Cover and refrigerate overnight.

4. Before serving, stir well and top with fresh berries.

Nutritional Facts (per serving):

- Calories: 130 kcal

- Protein: 4g

- Carbohydrates: 9g

- Fat: 8g

- Fiber: 8g

Gluten-Free Zucchini Fritters

- **Prep Time:** 10 minutes

- **Cook Time:** 15 minutes

- **Serving Size:** 4 servings

Ingredients:

- 2 medium zucchinis, grated

- 1/4 cup gluten-free flour

- 1 egg, beaten

- 1/4 cup green onions, chopped

- 1 garlic clove, minced

- Salt and pepper to taste

- 2 tablespoons olive oil

Instructions:

1. Place grated zucchini in a clean towel and squeeze out excess moisture.

2. In a bowl, combine zucchini, flour, egg, green onions, and garlic. Season with salt and pepper.

3. Heat olive oil in a large skillet over medium heat.

4. Drop spoonfuls of the mixture into the skillet and flatten with a spatula.

5. Cook for 3-4 minutes on each side, or until golden brown.

6. Serve warm.

Nutritional Facts (per serving):

- Calories: 150 kcal

- Protein: 4g

- Carbohydrates: 10g

- Fat: 11g

- Fiber: 2g

Dairy-Free Banana Ice Cream

- **Prep Time:** 5 minutes

- **Cook Time:** 0 minutes

- **Serving Size:** 2 servings

Ingredients:

- 3 ripe bananas, sliced and frozen

- 1 teaspoon vanilla extract

- 1 tablespoon almond butter (optional)

Instructions:

1. In a food processor, blend frozen banana slices until smooth.

2. Add vanilla extract and almond butter, if using. Blend until combined.

3. Serve immediately as soft-serve or freeze for 1-2 hours for a firmer texture.

Nutritional Facts (per serving):

- Calories: 120 kcal

- Protein: 1g

- Carbohydrates: 31g

- Fat: 0g

- Fiber: 3g

Vegan Lentil Stew

- **Prep Time:** 10 minutes

- **Cook Time:** 30 minutes

- **Serving Size:** 4 servings

Ingredients:

- 1 cup green or brown lentils

- 1 onion, chopped

- 2 carrots, diced

- 2 celery stalks, diced

- 3 garlic cloves, minced

- 4 cups vegetable broth

- 1 can diced tomatoes

- 1 teaspoon ground cumin

- 1 teaspoon smoked paprika

- Salt and pepper to taste

- 1 tablespoon olive oil

Instructions:

1. Heat olive oil in a large pot over medium heat. Add onion, carrots, and celery, and sauté until softened.

2. Add garlic and cook for another minute.

3. Stir in lentils, vegetable broth, diced tomatoes, cumin, and smoked paprika.

4. Bring to a boil, then reduce heat and simmer for 30 minutes, or until lentils are tender.

5. Season with salt and pepper to taste.

6. Serve hot.

Nutritional Facts (per serving):

- Calories: 220 kcal

- Protein: 12g

- Carbohydrates: 37g

- Fat: 3g

- Fiber: 15g

Low-Sugar Coconut Macaroons

- **Prep Time:** 10 minutes

- **Cook Time:** 20 minutes

- **Serving Size:** 12 macaroons

Ingredients:

- 2 cups unsweetened shredded coconut

- 1/4 cup coconut flour

- 1/4 cup coconut oil, melted

- 1/4 cup stevia or monk fruit sweetener

- 1 teaspoon vanilla extract

- Pinch of sea salt

Instructions:

1. Preheat oven to 325°F (165°C) and line a baking sheet with parchment paper.

2. In a bowl, mix all ingredients until well combined.

3. Scoop tablespoon-sized mounds onto the baking sheet.

4. Bake for 20 minutes or until golden brown.

5. Let cool before serving.

Nutritional Facts (per macaroon):

- Calories: 100 kcal

- Protein: 1g

- Carbohydrates: 5g

- Fat: 9g

- Fiber: 3g

Gluten-Free Sweet Potato Pancakes

- **Prep Time:** 10 minutes

- **Cook Time:** 10 minutes

- **Serving Size:** 4 servings

Ingredients:

- 1 large sweet potato, cooked and mashed

- 2 eggs

- 1/4 cup coconut flour

- 1 teaspoon cinnamon

- 1/4 teaspoon nutmeg

- 1/2 teaspoon baking soda

- Pinch of salt

- 2 tablespoons coconut oil

Instructions:

1. In a bowl, mix mashed sweet potato, eggs, coconut flour, cinnamon, nutmeg, baking soda, and salt until smooth.

2. Heat coconut oil in a skillet over medium heat.

3. Pour 1/4 cup of the batter into the skillet for each pancake.

4. Cook for 3-4 minutes on each side, or until golden brown.

5. Serve warm.

Nutritional Facts (per serving):

- Calories: 160 kcal

- Protein: 4g

- Carbohydrates: 18g

- Fat: 8g

- Fiber: 4g

Dairy-Free Green Smoothie Bowl

- **Prep Time:** 5 minutes

- **Cook Time:** 0 minutes

- **Serving Size:** 2 servings

Ingredients:

- 2 cups spinach

- 1 banana

- 1/2 avocado

- 1 cup unsweetened almond milk

- 1 tablespoon chia seeds

- Fresh berries and granola for topping

Instructions:

1. In a blender, combine spinach, banana, avocado, almond milk, and chia seeds.

2. Blend until smooth.

3. Pour into bowls and top with fresh berries and granola.

4. Serve immediately.

Nutritional Facts (per serving):

- Calories: 200 kcal

- Protein: 4g

- Carbohydrates: 27g

- Fat: 10g

- Fiber: 9g

Conclusion

Adopting an anti-inflammatory diet can lead to improved health and well-being. By focusing on full, nutrient-dense foods and eliminating potential dietary sources of inflammation, you can help manage and prevent chronic inflammation, which has been linked to a variety of health issues.

In this cookbook, we've included a selection of dishes tailored to varied nutritional needs while stressing anti-inflammatory elements. From hearty breakfasts to refreshing beverages, each recipe is designed to be both delicious and good for you.

As you continue your anti-inflammatory diet journey, keep in mind that the goal is to make long-term adjustments that work for you. Experiment with new ingredients and recipes, but most importantly, listen to your body. Your health is a lifetime endeavor, and every small step toward less inflammation counts.

We hope these recipes encourage you to discover the beautiful world of anti-inflammatory foods and help you become a healthier, more vibrant version of yourself. Here's to your health and culinary adventures!